THE NO-CARB FOOD LIST

A Step-By-Step Guide To Eliminating Carbs From Your Diet

Petra Kub

i

Table of Contents

Introduction

Are you looking to transform your diet and embrace healthier eating? If you've ever wondered about eliminating carbs from your meals, "The No-Carb Food List: A Step-by-Step Guide to Eliminating Carbs from Your Diet" is your ultimate resource. In this comprehensive guide, we'll take you on a journey to understand the impact of carbohydrates on your health and provide you with practical steps to transition to a no-carb lifestyle.

Carbohydrates, commonly found in foods like bread, pasta, and sugary treats, are a primary energy source for our bodies. However, not all carbs are created equal, and an excessive intake of refined carbohydrates can lead to various health issues, including weight gain, insulin resistance, and inflammation.

By understanding the different types of carbohydrates and their effects on your body, you'll be empowered to make informed decisions about your dietary choices. We aim to equip you with the knowledge to create a no-carb food list that includes nutritious and delicious alternatives, ensuring you never feel deprived or unsatisfied.

This guide'll explore the benefits and potential challenges of adopting a no-carb diet. The positive impacts can be life-changing, from weight loss and improved energy levels to mental clarity and enhanced focus. However, we'll also address common obstacles you may encounter during the transition and provide you with strategies to overcome them successfully.

A significant aspect of embarking on a no-carb journey involves mental and physical preparation. We'll guide you through setting realistic goals and developing a positive mindset to stay motivated. Additionally, we'll emphasize the importance of listening to your body and understanding its needs as you embark on this transformative dietary change.

Creating a variety of delicious no-carb meals is at the heart of this guide. From mouthwatering breakfast options to satisfying lunches and dinners, we'll present various flavorful choices. Say goodbye to carb-heavy favorites like sandwiches and pasta, and say hello to creative and nutrient-rich meals that will keep you energized and content throughout the day.

Social situations and dining out can be challenging on a no-carb diet. However, armed with the knowledge and confidence gained from this guide, you'll be prepared to easily navigate these situations, ensuring you stick to your dietary goals without feeling isolated or restricted.

Adopting a no-carb lifestyle is a personal journey, and it's essential to approach it with balance and mindfulness. Before making any significant changes to your diet, we encourage you to consult a healthcare professional to ensure it aligns with your needs and health status.

Let's embark on this exciting adventure together as we explore the world of no-carb living and pave the way for a healthier and happier you!

Understanding Carbohydrates and Their Impact on Your Health

This section delves deep into carbohydrates and their significant impact on your health. Carbohydrates, commonly called "carbs," are one of the three macronutrients in our diet, alongside proteins and fats. They are vital in providing energy to our bodies, but not all carbohydrates are created equal. Understanding the different types of carbs and how they affect your health is essential in making informed choices about your dietary intake.

Types of Carbohydrates

Carbohydrates can be broadly categorized into two main types: simple carbohydrates and complex carbohydrates. Simple carbohydrates consist of one or two sugar molecules and are quickly digested, leading to a rapid spike in blood sugar levels. Examples of simple carbs include table sugar, candy, soda, and processed foods. On the other hand, complex carbohydrates comprise multiple sugar molecules and take longer to digest, providing a more sustained release of energy. Foods rich in complex carbs include whole grains, vegetables, legumes, and fruits.

Blood Sugar and Insulin Response

When you consume carbohydrates, they are broken down into glucose, which enters your bloodstream. The rise in blood sugar triggers the release of insulin, a hormone produced by the pancreas. Insulin helps transport glucose from the bloodstream into the cells, which can be used for energy. However, excessive consumption of simple carbohydrates can lead to frequent spikes in blood sugar levels, causing the pancreas to overwork insulin production. Over time, this can lead to insulin resistance, a condition where the cells become less responsive to insulin, increasing the risk of type 2 diabetes.

Carbohydrates and Weight Management

The relationship between carbohydrates and weight management has been debated for years. Some diets advocate drastically reducing carbohydrate intake, while others focus on moderation and balance. The truth lies in understanding the quality and quantity of carbs you consume. Simple carbs with empty calories, such as sugary beverages and refined snacks, can contribute to weight gain and hinder weight loss efforts. On the other hand, consuming complex carbs and a balanced diet can promote satiety, helping you feel full for longer and prevent overeating.

The Glycemic Index (GI)

The glycemic index (GI) is a scale that ranks carbohydrates based on how quickly they raise blood sugar levels. Foods with a high GI, such as white bread and sugary cereals, cause rapid spikes in blood sugar, while low-GI foods, like sweet potatoes and quinoa, lead to a slower and more gradual increase. Incorporating more low-GI foods into your diet can help regulate blood sugar levels, improve insulin sensitivity, and aid in weight management.

Carbohydrates and Gut Health

Carbohydrates also play a crucial role in maintaining a healthy gut. Certain types of carbohydrates, known as prebiotics, act as food for beneficial gut bacteria. These bacteria help digest fiber and produce short-chain fatty acids essential for gut health and overall well-being. Foods like onions, garlic, asparagus, and bananas are rich sources of prebiotics and can contribute to a balanced gut microbiome.

Carbohydrates and Exercise

Carbohydrates are the primary fuel source for high-intensity exercise and athletic performance. When you engage in intense physical activity, your body relies on glycogen, the stored form of glucose, to sustain energy levels. A well-balanced diet with sufficient complex carbohydrates is crucial for athletes and active individuals to enhance performance and promote optimal recovery.

Moderation and Balance

While there are valid concerns about the overconsumption of refined carbohydrates and their impact on health, it's essential to remember that not all carbohydrates are harmful. Carbohydrates are vital to a healthy diet and should be consumed in moderation and balance. Eliminating all carbs from your diet may not be sustainable or practical, as many nutritious and beneficial foods fall under this category. The key is to focus on whole, unprocessed foods and choose complex carbs that provide lasting energy and essential nutrients.

Benefits and Challenges of a No-Carb Diet

Here, we will delve into the world of no-carb diets, exploring their potential benefits for your health and well-being. A no-carb diet, a low-carb or ketogenic diet, involves significantly reducing or eliminating carbohydrates from your daily meals. This approach aims to shift your body's primary fuel source from carbohydrates to fats, leading to physiological changes and potential health advantages. However, like any dietary change, a no-carb diet has challenges that must be considered before embarking on this transformative journey.

Benefits of a No-Carb Diet

Weight Loss and Improved Body Composition

One of the primary reasons people turn to a no-carb diet is its potential to promote weight loss. By reducing carb intake, the body enters ketosis, burning stored fats for energy instead of relying on carbohydrates. This shift in fuel source can lead to more efficient fat burning, resulting in weight loss and improved body composition. Several studies have shown that low-carb diets can be more effective for weight loss than low-fat diets, especially in the short term.

Stable Blood Sugar Levels

For individuals with diabetes or insulin resistance, a no-carb diet can be particularly beneficial. By minimizing carbohydrate intake, blood sugar levels remain more stable, reducing the need for frequent insulin spikes. This can lead to better glycemic control and help manage diabetes more effectively.

Enhanced Mental Clarity and Focus

Some individuals report improved mental clarity and focus when following a no-carb diet. Ketones, produced during ketosis, serve as an alternative energy source for the brain and may provide a steady fuel supply, resulting in increased cognitive function and mental acuity.

Reduced Hunger and Appetite

Many people find that a no-carb diet helps control hunger and appetite. High-carb meals can lead to rapid spikes and crashes in blood sugar levels, triggering feelings of hunger and cravings. By adopting a no-carb approach, you may experience more stable energy levels and feel satiated for extended periods, reducing the likelihood of overeating.

Improved Cardiovascular Health

Research suggests that a no-carb diet may positively impact cardiovascular risk factors, such as reducing triglycerides, increasing HDL (good) cholesterol levels, and improving blood pressure. However, it's essential to focus on healthy fats and avoid excessive saturated and trans fats to maximize these benefits.

Challenges of a No-Carb Diet

Keto Flu and Initial Side Effects

When transitioning to a no-carb diet, some individuals may experience what is commonly known as the "keto flu." This temporary phase may include symptoms like headache, fatigue, dizziness, and irritability as the body adapts to using fats as its primary fuel source. While these side effects are typically short-lived, they can be challenging to endure during the initial stages of the diet.

Nutrient Deficiencies

Eliminating or significantly reducing certain food groups, such as fruits, whole grains, and legumes, can lead to potential nutrient deficiencies. These food items are rich in essential vitamins, minerals, and dietary fiber that contribute to overall health. It's essential to carefully plan a no-carb diet to ensure you still get all the necessary nutrients through other food sources or supplementation.

Social Challenges and Dining Out

Following a no-carb diet can be socially challenging, especially during gatherings or dining out. Many traditional social settings involve carb-heavy dishes, and finding suitable no-carb alternatives can be tricky. This may lead to feelings of isolation or temptation to stray from the diet.

Digestive Issues

For some individuals, consuming large amounts of fats and proteins while significantly reducing carbohydrates can cause digestive discomfort. Typical issues may include constipation, bloating, and indigestion. Ensuring you're incorporating enough fiber from non-starchy vegetables and staying hydrated can help mitigate these problems.

Long-Term Sustainability

The strict nature of a no-carb diet can be challenging for some individuals to maintain in the long term. Excluding certain foods may lead to cravings and feelings of deprivation, potentially making it difficult to sustain the diet over extended periods.

Preparing Yourself Mentally and Physically for the No-Carb Journey

Embarking on a no-carb journey requires more than just changing your dietary habits. It involves preparing yourself mentally and physically for the challenges and changes ahead. This section will guide you through getting ready for the no-carb lifestyle, ensuring you have the right mindset and tools to succeed on this transformative path.

Setting Realistic Goals

Before diving into a no-carb diet, setting realistic and achievable goals is crucial. Define what you want to accomplish with this dietary change, and be specific about your intentions. Whether it's weight loss, improved energy levels, or better blood sugar control, clear goals will provide you with direction and motivation throughout your journey. For example, instead of a vague goal like "lose weight," set a specific target, such as "lose 10 pounds in three months," which is measurable and attainable.

11

Educate Yourself

Knowledge is power, especially when it comes to understanding the no-carb lifestyle. Educate yourself about the science behind a no-carb diet, how it affects your body, and the potential benefits and challenges you may encounter. Read books, watch documentaries, and seek reputable online sources to gather information. Understanding the reasoning behind this dietary choice will help you stay committed and confident in your decision.

Identify Triggers and Challenges

Take time to identify your triggers and potential challenges regarding your dietary habits. Are there specific carb-rich foods you find hard to resist? Are there emotional or social situations that lead to overindulgence in carbohydrates? By recognizing these triggers, you can develop strategies to overcome them and stay on track with your no-carb goals. For instance, if stress triggers emotional eating, find alternative coping mechanisms like meditation or exercise.

Build a Support System

Having a supportive network of friends, family, or like-minded individuals can significantly impact your success on a no-carb diet. Share your goals and journey with them, and consider finding a buddy or joining a community following a no-carb lifestyle. Having people who understand and encourage your choices will provide accountability and motivation during challenging times.

Gradual Transition

If you're used to a carbohydrate-rich diet, suddenly eliminating them can shock your system. Consider gradually transitioning to a no-carb diet to allow your body to adapt slowly. Start by reducing refined carbs and sugary treats, and gradually increase your consumption of non-starchy vegetables, healthy fats, and proteins. This gradual approach can minimize potential side effects and make the adjustment more manageable.

Mindful Eating

Practicing mindful eating is essential in any dietary change. Pay attention to your hunger and fullness cues, and eat with intention and awareness. Slow down during meals, savor each bite, and stop eating when satisfied. Mindful eating can help prevent overeating and enhance your overall eating experience.

Prepare Your Kitchen

Preparing your kitchen for a no-carb lifestyle is crucial in ensuring success. Remove carb-heavy foods from your pantry and replace them with no-carb alternatives. Stock up on fresh vegetables, lean proteins, healthy fats, and low-carb snacks to have readily available. A well-prepared kitchen will make it easier to stick to your dietary plan and avoid temptations.

Stay Positive and Flexible

As you embark on your no-carb journey, maintain a positive attitude and be open to flexibility. There may be moments when you deviate from your diet, and that's okay. Instead of viewing it as a failure, see it as an opportunity to learn and grow. Stay focused on your long-term goals, and don't let occasional slip-ups derail your progress.

Creating Your No-Carb Food List and Meal Planning

Now that you're mentally and physically prepared for the no-carb journey, it's time to dive into the heart of your dietary transformation – creating a no-carb food list and mastering the art of meal planning. In this section, we'll guide you through curating a well-balanced and delicious no-carb food list, ensuring you have a diverse range of nutrient-rich options. Additionally, we'll explore the art of meal planning, helping you prepare satisfying and wholesome meals that align with your no-carb goals.

The No-Carb Food List

Non-Starchy Vegetables

Non-starchy vegetables will become the foundation of your no-carb food list. These vegetables are low in carbohydrates and calories but rich in essential vitamins, minerals, and fiber. Examples include leafy greens (spinach, kale, arugula), broccoli, cauliflower, zucchini, bell peppers, asparagus, and mushrooms. These vegetables provide vital nutrients and add texture and flavor to your meals.

Proteins

Proteins are essential for maintaining muscle mass, supporting immune function, and providing satiety. Opt for high-quality, lean sources of protein that are low in carbohydrates. Some excellent options include poultry (chicken, turkey), seafood (salmon, tuna, shrimp), lean cuts of beef and pork, eggs, and plant-based proteins like tofu and tempeh. When choosing processed meats like bacon or sausages, check for hidden carbohydrates in the form of added sugars or fillers.

Healthy Fats

Healthy fats are a valuable energy source on a no-carb diet and play a crucial role in various bodily functions. Incorporate sources of healthy fats such as avocados, nuts (almonds, walnuts, macadamia nuts), seeds (chia seeds, flaxseeds), and olive oil.

Fats not only add richness to your meals but also help keep you feeling full and satisfied.

Dairy

Dairy products can be included in a no-carb diet, but it's essential to choose wisely. Opt for full-fat and unsweetened options to minimize carbohydrate intake. Examples include whole milk, plain Greek yogurt, and cheese. Some individuals may need to limit dairy consumption due to lactose intolerance, so be mindful of how your body responds to dairy products.

Low-Carb Fruits

While many fruits are naturally high in carbohydrates, some can be enjoyed in moderation on a no-carb diet. Berries, such as strawberries, raspberries, and blackberries, are lower in carbs and rich in antioxidants and fiber. Just be mindful of portion sizes to avoid consuming too many carbs from fruits.

Mastering Meal Planning

Plan Ahead

Start your week with a meal planning session. Plan your meals for the upcoming days, considering your schedule, dietary preferences, and the ingredients you have on hand. A well-thought-out plan will save you time and make grocery shopping more efficient.

Batch Cooking

Consider batch-cooking specific components of your meals to save time and ensure you always have nutritious options available. For example, cook a batch of grilled chicken, roasted vegetables, or cauliflower rice that can be used in various dishes throughout the week.

Balance Your Meals

Aim for balanced meals that include a source of protein, healthy fats, and non-starchy vegetables. A typical no-carb meal could be grilled salmon with steamed broccoli and avocado sliced with olive oil.

Embrace No-Carb Substitutes

Get creative with no-carb substitutes for your favorite carb-heavy dishes. For example, use zucchini noodles or "zoodles" instead of pasta, cauliflower rice instead of regular rice, or lettuce wraps instead of tortillas.

Snack Smartly

Having no-carb snacks on hand can help curb hunger between meals. Prepare snacks like cucumber slices with cream cheese, celery sticks with almond butter, or a handful of mixed nuts to satisfy you throughout the day.

No-Carb Breakfasts to Kickstart Your Day

Breakfast is often hailed as the most important meal of the day, and on a no-carb diet, it becomes an excellent opportunity to energize your body and fuel it with nutrient-rich foods. In this section, we'll explore various delicious and satisfying no-carb breakfast options that will kickstart your day on a healthy note. From savory omelets to delightful smoothies, these recipes will ensure you never miss those carb-heavy breakfast staples.

Veggie and Cheese Omelet

Ingredients:

- 3 large eggs
- 1/4 cup diced bell peppers (any color)
- 1/4 cup diced onions
- 1/4 cup diced tomatoes
- 1/4 cup shredded cheddar cheese
- Salt and pepper to taste
- 1 tablespoon olive oil
1. Instructions:

2. In a bowl, whisk the eggs and season with salt and pepper.
3. Heat the olive oil in a non-stick skillet over medium heat.
4. Add the diced bell peppers and onions to the skillet and sauté until softened.
5. Pour the whisked eggs into the skillet, ensuring they spread evenly to cover the veggies.
6. Cook the omelet for 2-3 minutes or until the edges are set.
7. Sprinkle the diced tomatoes and shredded cheddar cheese over one-half of the omelet.
8. Carefully fold the other half of the omelet over the filling, creating a half-moon shape.
9. Cook for another 1-2 minutes until the cheese is melted and the omelet is fully set.
10. Slide the omelet onto a plate and serve hot.

Nutrition (per serving):
- Calories: 350
- Carbohydrates: 7g

- Protein: 23g
- Fat: 26g
- Fiber: 2g

Creamy Avocado and Spinach Smoothie

Ingredients:

- 1 ripe avocado, pitted and peeled
- 1 cup fresh spinach leaves
- 1 cup unsweetened almond milk
- 1 tablespoon almond butter
- 1 tablespoon chia seeds
- 1 teaspoon honey (optional, for sweetness)
- Ice cubes (optional, for a chilled smoothie)

Instructions:

1. Combine the avocado, spinach, almond milk, almond butter, chia seeds, and honey (if using).
2. Blend until smooth and creamy.
3. If you prefer a chilled smoothie, add some ice cubes to the blender and blend until well combined.

4. Pour the smoothie into a glass and enjoy immediately.

Nutrition (per serving):

- Calories: 300
- Carbohydrates: 12g
- Protein: 6g
- Fat: 25g
- Fiber: 8g

Smoked Salmon and Avocado Wrap

Ingredients:

- 2 large lettuce leaves (butter lettuce or romaine work well)
- 2 ounces smoked salmon
- 1/2 avocado, sliced
- 1 tablespoon cream cheese
- 1 teaspoon capers (optional, for added flavor)
- Fresh dill (for garnish)

Instructions:

1. Lay the lettuce leaves on a clean surface.

2. Spread the cream cheese evenly on each lettuce leaf.
3. Place the smoked salmon on top of the cream cheese.
4. Add the sliced avocado and sprinkle capers over the filling.
5. Garnish with fresh dill.
6. Carefully roll up the lettuce leaves to form a wrap.
7. Secure with toothpicks if needed.
8. Serve the smoked salmon and avocado wrap as a refreshing, no-carb breakfast option.

Nutrition (per serving):

- Calories: 250
- Carbohydrates: 5g
- Protein: 15g
- Fat: 18g
- Fiber: 3g

Mushroom and Spinach Frittata

Ingredients:

- 6 large eggs

- 1 cup sliced mushrooms
- 1 cup fresh spinach leaves
- 1/4 cup shredded mozzarella cheese
- 1 tablespoon olive oil
- Salt and pepper to taste

Instructions:

1. Preheat the oven to 350°F (175°C).
2. In an oven-safe skillet, heat the olive oil over medium heat.
3. Add the sliced mushrooms and sauté until they release moisture and become tender.
4. Add the fresh spinach leaves to the skillet and cook until wilted.
5. In a bowl, whisk the eggs and season with salt and pepper.
6. Pour the whisked eggs into the skillet, evenly covering the mushrooms and spinach.
7. Sprinkle shredded mozzarella cheese over the frittata.
8. Transfer the skillet to the preheated oven and bake for 12-15 minutes or until the eggs are fully set.

9. Remove from the oven and let it cool slightly before slicing and serving.

Nutrition (per serving):

- Calories: 280
- Carbohydrates: 5g
- Protein: 20g
- Fat: 20g
- Fiber: 1g

Mushroom and Spinach Frittata

Ingredients:

- 6 large eggs
- 1 cup sliced mushrooms
- 1 cup fresh spinach leaves
- 1/4 cup shredded mozzarella cheese
- 1 tablespoon olive oil
- Salt and pepper to taste

Instructions:

1. Preheat the oven to 350°F (175°C).
2. In an oven-safe skillet, heat the olive oil over medium heat.

3. Add the sliced mushrooms and sauté until they release moisture and become tender.
4. Add the fresh spinach leaves to the skillet and cook until wilted.
5. In a bowl, whisk the eggs and season with salt and pepper.
6. Pour the whisked eggs into the skillet, evenly covering the mushrooms and spinach.
7. Sprinkle shredded mozzarella cheese over the frittata.
8. Transfer the skillet to the preheated oven and bake for 12-15 minutes or until the eggs are fully set.
9. Remove from the oven and let it cool slightly before slicing and serving.

Nutrition (per serving):
- Calories: 280
- Carbohydrates: 5g
- Protein: 20g
- Fat: 20g
- Fiber: 1g

Greek Yogurt Parfait with Berries and Nuts

Ingredients:

- 1 cup plain Greek yogurt
- 1/2 cup mixed berries (strawberries, blueberries, raspberries)
- 2 tablespoons chopped nuts (almonds, walnuts)
- 1 tablespoon chia seeds
- 1 teaspoon honey (optional, for added sweetness)

Instructions:

1. Layer the Greek yogurt, mixed berries, chopped nuts, and chia seeds in a serving glass or bowl.
2. Drizzle honey over the top for added sweetness, if desired.
3. Repeat the layers to create a visually appealing and nutritious parfait.
4. Serve immediately or refrigerate for a relaxed and refreshing breakfast option.

Nutrition (per serving):

- Calories: 300
- Carbohydrates: 15g
- Protein: 20g
- Fat: 18g
- Fiber: 6g

No-Carb Breakfast Burrito Bowl

Ingredients:

- 4 large eggs
- 1/2 cup diced bell peppers (any color)
- 1/2 cup diced onions
- 1/2 cup diced tomatoes
- 1/4 cup sliced black olives
- 1/4 cup shredded cheddar cheese
- 1 tablespoon olive oil
- Salt and pepper to taste
- Fresh cilantro (for garnish)

Instructions:

1. In a skillet, heat the olive oil over medium heat.
2. Add the diced bell peppers and onions to the skillet and sauté until softened.

3. Crack the eggs directly into the skillet, ensuring they are evenly distributed among the veggies.
4. Scramble the eggs with the vegetables until fully cooked.
5. Season with salt and pepper to taste.
6. Transfer the scrambled eggs and veggies to a serving bowl.
7. Top with diced tomatoes, sliced black olives, and shredded cheddar cheese.
8. Garnish with fresh cilantro for added flavor and a pop of color.
9. Mix all the ingredients in the bowl, and your no-carb breakfast burrito bowl is ready to enjoy.

Nutrition (per serving):
- Calories: 350
- Carbohydrates: 7g
- Protein: 21g
- Fat: 26g
- Fiber: 2g

Delicious and Filling No-Carb Lunch Ideas

Lunchtime allows you to refuel your body and continue your no-carb journey with mouthwatering and satisfying meals. In this section, we'll explore various delicious no-carb lunch ideas that will keep you feeling full and nourished throughout the day. From hearty salads to flavorful wraps, these recipes will not only tantalize your taste buds but also support your health and well-being.

Grilled Chicken Salad with Avocado Dressing

Ingredients:

- 4 ounces grilled chicken breast, sliced
- 2 cups mixed salad greens (lettuce, spinach, arugula)
- 1/2 avocado, diced
- 1/4 cup cherry tomatoes, halved
- 1/4 cup cucumber slices
- 1 tablespoon pumpkin seeds
- 2 tablespoons olive oil
- 1 tablespoon lemon juice

- Salt and pepper to taste

Instructions:

1. Combine the mixed salad greens, diced avocado, cherry tomatoes, and cucumber slices in a large bowl.
2. Top the salad with sliced grilled chicken.
3. Whisk together olive oil, lemon juice, salt, and pepper in a small bowl to create the avocado dressing.
4. Drizzle the avocado dressing over the salad.
5. Sprinkle pumpkin seeds over the top for added crunch and nutrition.
6. Toss the salad gently to coat all the ingredients with the dressing.
7. Transfer to a serving plate and enjoy your refreshing and filling no-carb lunch.

Nutrition (per serving):

- Calories: 400
- Carbohydrates: 9g
- Protein: 25g
- Fat: 30g

- Fiber: 5g

Cauliflower Rice Stir-Fry

Ingredients:

- 1 cup cauliflower rice
- 4 ounces cooked shrimp or tofu (for a vegetarian option)
- 1/2 cup broccoli florets
- 1/4 cup sliced bell peppers (any color)
- 1/4 cup sliced carrots
- 2 tablespoons soy sauce (or tamari for a gluten-free option)
- 1 tablespoon sesame oil
- 1 teaspoon minced garlic
- 1 teaspoon grated ginger
- 1 tablespoon chopped green onions (for garnish)
- Sesame seeds (for garnish)

Instructions:

1. Heat the sesame oil over medium heat in a wok or large skillet.

2. Add the minced garlic, grated ginger, and sauté until fragrant.
3. Add the sliced bell peppers and carrots to the wok, and stir-fry for 2-3 minutes until slightly softened.
4. Add the cauliflower rice and broccoli florets to the wok and stir-fry for another 2-3 minutes until the cauliflower is tender.
5. Stir in the cooked shrimp or tofu, and drizzle soy sauce over the stir-fry, tossing to coat all the ingredients evenly.
6. Cook for 1-2 minutes until everything is heated and well combined.
7. Transfer the cauliflower rice stir-fry to a serving dish.
8. Garnish with chopped green onions and sesame seeds for added flavor and visual appeal.
9. Serve hot and savor the flavors of this delightful no-carb lunch.

Nutrition (per serving):

- Calories: 350
- Carbohydrates: 12g
- Protein: 20g
- Fat: 25g
- Fiber: 5g

Zucchini Noodle Chicken Alfredo

Ingredients:

- 1 large zucchini, spiralized into noodles
- 4 ounces grilled chicken breast, sliced
- 1/4 cup heavy cream
- 2 tablespoons grated parmesan cheese
- 1 tablespoon butter
- 1 teaspoon minced garlic
- Salt and pepper to taste
- Fresh parsley (for garnish)

Instructions:

1. In a saucepan, melt the butter over medium heat.
2. Add the minced garlic to the saucepan, and sauté for a minute until fragrant.

36

3. Stir in the heavy cream and grated parmesan cheese, cooking until the cheese is melted and the sauce thickens.
4. Season the sauce with salt and pepper to taste.
5. Add the zucchini noodles to the saucepan, tossing them in the alfredo sauce to coat evenly.
6. Cook for 2-3 minutes until the zucchini noodles are heated through.
7. Top the zucchini noodle alfredo with sliced grilled chicken.
8. Garnish with fresh parsley for a burst of color and freshness.
9. Serve immediately and indulge in this creamy and no-carb lunch delight.

Nutrition (per serving):
- Calories: 380
- Carbohydrates: 10g
- Protein: 30g
- Fat: 25g
- Fiber: 2g

Turkey and Avocado Lettuce Wraps

Ingredients:

- 4 large lettuce leaves (iceberg or butter lettuce work well)
- 4 ounces deli turkey slices (choose no-carb or low-carb options)
- 1/2 avocado, sliced
- 1/4 cup shredded carrots
- 1/4 cup sliced cucumbers
- 2 tablespoons hummus (for added creaminess, choose a no-carb or low-carb version)

Instructions:

1. Lay the lettuce leaves on a clean surface.
2. Spread hummus evenly on each lettuce leaf.
3. Layer the deli turkey, avocado, shredded carrots, and cucumber slices over the hummus.
4. Carefully roll up the lettuce leaves to form wraps.
5. Secure with toothpicks if needed.

6. Serve the turkey and avocado lettuce wraps as a no-carb lunch option that's refreshing and satisfying.

Nutrition (per serving):
- Calories: 300
- Carbohydrates: 10g
- Protein: 18g
- Fat: 20g
- Fiber: 5g

Caprese Stuffed Portobello Mushrooms

Ingredients:
- 2 large Portobello mushrooms
- 4 slices fresh mozzarella cheese
- 1 cup cherry tomatoes, halved
- 1/4 cup fresh basil leaves
- 2 tablespoons balsamic glaze
- 2 tablespoons olive oil
- Salt and pepper to taste

Instructions:

1. Preheat the oven to 400°F (200°C).
2. Clean the Portobello mushrooms and remove the stems.
3. Brush the mushrooms with olive oil on both sides and season with salt and pepper.
4. Place the mushrooms on a baking sheet, gill-side up.
5. Layer two slices of fresh mozzarella cheese on each mushroom.
6. Add the halved cherry tomatoes on top of the cheese.
7. Bake in the oven for 12-15 minutes or until the cheese is melted and bubbly.
8. Remove the stuffed mushrooms from the oven and garnish with fresh basil leaves.
9. Drizzle balsamic glaze over the top for a tangy and sweet finish.
10. Serve the Caprese stuffed Portobello mushrooms as a delightful no-carb dinner option.

Nutrition (per serving):

- Calories: 300
- Carbohydrates: 10g
- Protein: 15g
- Fat: 20g
- Fiber: 3g

Lemon Garlic Butter Shrimp

Ingredients:

- 1 pound large shrimp, peeled and deveined
- 3 tablespoons butter
- 3 cloves garlic, minced
- Juice of 1 lemon
- Zest of 1 lemon
- 2 tablespoons chopped fresh parsley
- Salt and pepper to taste

Instructions:

1. In a large skillet, melt the butter over medium heat.
2. Add the minced garlic to the skillet and sauté until fragrant.

3. Add the shrimp to the skillet and cook on each side for 2-3 minutes until they turn pink and opaque.
4. Stir in the lemon juice and zest, and season with salt and pepper to taste.
5. Cook for another minute to allow the flavors to meld.
6. Sprinkle chopped fresh parsley over the shrimp for added freshness and color.
7. Serve the lemon garlic butter shrimp as a delightful, flavorful, no-carb dinner option.

Nutrition (per serving):

- Calories: 250
- Carbohydrates: 3g
- Protein: 30g
- Fat: 12g
- Fiber: 0g

Stuffed Bell Peppers with Ground Beef and Cauliflower Rice

Ingredients:

- 4 large bell peppers (any color), tops removed and seeds discarded
- 1 pound ground beef (or turkey for a leaner option)
- 1 cup cauliflower rice
- 1 cup diced tomatoes (canned or fresh)
- 1/2 cup diced onions
- 2 cloves garlic, minced
- 1 tablespoon olive oil
- 1 teaspoon dried oregano
- 1 teaspoon dried basil
- Salt and pepper to taste
- 1/4 cup shredded mozzarella cheese (optional, for added indulgence)

Instructions:

1. Preheat the oven to 375°F (190°C).
2. In a large skillet, heat the olive oil over medium heat.

3. Add the diced onions and minced garlic to the skillet and sauté until softened.

4. Add the ground beef (or turkey) to the skillet and cook until browned and cooked through.

5. Stir in the diced tomatoes, cauliflower rice, dried oregano, dried basil, salt, and pepper, and cook for another 3-4 minutes to allow the flavors to meld.

6. Stuff each bell pepper with the ground beef and cauliflower rice mixture, pressing it down gently to fill each pepper evenly.

7. Place the stuffed bell peppers on a baking sheet and bake in the oven for 25-30 minutes or until the peppers are tender.

8. If desired, sprinkle shredded mozzarella cheese over the stuffed peppers during the last 5 minutes of baking for a cheesy and indulgent finish.

9. Remove the stuffed bell peppers from the oven and let them cool slightly before serving.

Nutrition (per serving):

- Calories: 350
- Carbohydrates: 12g
- Protein: 25g
- Fat: 20g
- Fiber: 4g

Satisfying No-Carb Dinners for a Healthy Lifestyle

As the day ends, it's time to end with a satisfying and wholesome no-carb dinner. This section explores delectable no-carb dinner recipes that will nourish your body and support your commitment to a healthy lifestyle. From hearty meat dishes to delightful vegetarian options, these dinners are designed to keep you full, satisfied, and energized.

Grilled Steak with Garlic Butter

Ingredients:

- 8-ounce steak (choose your favorite cut)
- 2 tablespoons butter, softened
- 2 cloves garlic, minced
- 1 tablespoon chopped fresh parsley
- Salt and pepper to taste

Instructions:

1. Preheat the grill to medium-high heat.
2. Season the steak with salt and pepper on both sides.
3. Place the steak on the grill and cook to your desired level of doneness. (For a medium-

rare steak, cook for 4-5 minutes on each side.)

4. While the steak is grilling, prepare the garlic butter. Mix the softened butter, minced garlic, and chopped fresh parsley in a small bowl.

5. Once the steak is done, please remove it from the grill and rest for a few minutes.

6. Top the grilled steak with a generous dollop of garlic butter.

7. Serve the steak with no-carb side dishes, such as a Caesar salad or sautéed green beans.

Nutrition (per serving):
- Calories: 400
- Carbohydrates: 0g
- Protein: 30g
- Fat: 32g
- Fiber: 0g

Cauliflower Crust Pizza

Ingredients:

For the cauliflower crust:

- 1 medium cauliflower head, riced (about 2 cups)
- 1 large egg, beaten
- 1/2 cup shredded mozzarella cheese
- 1 teaspoon dried oregano
- 1/2 teaspoon garlic powder
- Salt and pepper to taste

For the pizza toppings:

- 1/2 cup sugar-free tomato sauce or pizza sauce
- 1/2 cup shredded mozzarella cheese
- Your favorite pizza toppings (e.g., pepperoni, mushrooms, bell peppers, olives)

Instructions:

1. Preheat the oven to 425°F (220°C).
2. Rice the cauliflower in a food processor or grate it using a box grater until it resembles rice grains.

3. Place the riced cauliflower in a microwave-safe bowl and microwave on high for 4-5 minutes until it's cooked.

4. Let the cooked cauliflower cool slightly, then transfer it to a clean kitchen towel. Squeeze out as much excess moisture as possible from the cauliflower.

5. Combine the cauliflower with the beaten egg, shredded mozzarella cheese, dried oregano, garlic powder, salt, and pepper in a bowl. Mix until well combined.

6. Line a baking sheet with parchment paper and spread the cauliflower mixture into a thin, even layer to form a pizza crust.

7. Bake the crust in the oven for 12-15 minutes, or until it's golden and holds together.

8. Remove the crust from the oven and add your pizza toppings – tomato sauce, shredded mozzarella cheese, and your favorite toppings.

9. Return the pizza to the oven and bake for another 8-10 minutes or until the cheese is melted and bubbly.
10. Let the cauliflower crust pizza cool slightly before slicing and serving.

Nutrition (per serving, based on crust only):

- Calories: 200
- Carbohydrates: 8g
- Protein: 12g
- Fat: 12g
- Fiber: 3g

Baked Lemon Herb Salmon

Ingredients:

- 4 salmon fillets
- 2 tablespoons olive oil
- 1 lemon, juiced and zested
- 2 cloves garlic, minced
- 1 tablespoon chopped fresh dill
- Salt and pepper to taste

Instructions:

1. Preheat the oven to 375°F (190°C).
2. Whisk together the olive oil, lemon juice, lemon zest, minced garlic, chopped dill, salt, and pepper in a small bowl.
3. Place the salmon fillets on a baking sheet lined with parchment paper.
4. Pour the lemon herb mixture over the salmon fillets, ensuring they are well coated on both sides.
5. Bake the salmon in the oven for 12-15 minutes or until it's cooked and flakes easily with a fork.
6. Remove the salmon from the oven and let it rest for a minute before serving.

Nutrition (per serving):

- Calories: 350
- Carbohydrates: 0g
- Protein: 35g
- Fat: 22g
- Fiber: 0g

Eggplant Parmesan

Ingredients:

- 1 large eggplant, sliced into rounds
- 1 cup almond flour (or almond meal)
- 1/2 cup grated parmesan cheese
- 2 large eggs, beaten
- 1 cup sugar-free tomato sauce
- 1 cup shredded mozzarella cheese
- 1/4 cup chopped fresh basil
- Salt and pepper to taste
- Olive oil (for frying)

Instructions:

1. Preheat the oven to 375°F (190°C).
2. In a shallow dish, mix the almond flour and grated parmesan cheese.
3. Dip each eggplant round into the beaten eggs, then coat it with the almond flour mixture, pressing it onto the eggplant to adhere.
4. In a large skillet, heat olive oil over medium heat. Fry the coated eggplant rounds in

batches until golden and crispy on both sides. Transfer them to a paper towel-lined plate to remove excess oil.

5. In a baking dish, spread a thin layer of tomato sauce on the bottom. Arrange a layer of fried eggplant rounds on top.

6. Sprinkle shredded mozzarella cheese and chopped basil over the eggplant layer.

7. Repeat the layers until all the eggplant is used, finishing with a layer of tomato sauce and mozzarella cheese.

8. Bake the eggplant Parmesan in the oven for 20-25 minutes or until the cheese is melted and bubbly.

9. Let it cool slightly before serving.

Nutrition (per serving):

- Calories: 300
- Carbohydrates: 8g
- Protein: 18g
- Fat: 22g
- Fiber: 4g

Zoodles with Pesto and Grilled Chicken

Ingredients:

- 2 medium zucchinis, spiralized into zoodles
- 2 boneless, skinless chicken breasts
- 1 cup fresh basil leaves
- 1/4 cup pine nuts
- 1/4 cup grated parmesan cheese
- 2 cloves garlic
- 1/2 cup olive oil
- Juice of 1 lemon
- Salt and pepper to taste

Instructions:

1. Preheat the grill to medium-high heat.
2. Season the chicken breasts with salt and pepper on both sides.
3. Grill the chicken for 6-7 minutes on each side or until it's cooked through and has grill marks. Let it rest for a few minutes before slicing.
4. While the chicken is grilling, prepare the pesto sauce. Combine the basil leaves, pine

nuts, grated parmesan cheese, garlic, and lemon juice in a food processor. Pulse until finely chopped.

5. Slowly drizzle in the olive oil with the food processor running until the pesto reaches your desired consistency - season with salt and pepper to taste.

6. Heat a tablespoon of olive oil over medium heat in a large skillet. Add the zoodles and cook for 2-3 minutes until they're slightly softened but still al dente.

7. Toss the zoodles with the pesto sauce until well coated.

8. Serve the zoodles with grilled chicken on top, and garnish with extra basil leaves and grated parmesan cheese.

Nutrition (per serving):

- Calories: 450
- Carbohydrates: 8g
- Protein: 35g
- Fat: 30g
- Fiber: 3g

Stuffed Bell Peppers with Quinoa and Black Beans

Ingredients:

- 4 large bell peppers (any color), tops removed and seeds discarded
- 1 cup cooked quinoa
- 1 cup cooked black beans
- 1 cup diced tomatoes (canned or fresh)
- 1/2 cup diced onions
- 1 teaspoon ground cumin
- 1 teaspoon chili powder
- Salt and pepper to taste
- 1/2 cup shredded cheddar cheese (optional, for topping)

Instructions:

1. Preheat the oven to 375°F (190°C).
2. In a large bowl, combine the cooked quinoa, cooked black beans, diced tomatoes, diced onions, ground cumin, chili powder, salt, and pepper.
3. Mix everything until well combined.

4. Stuff each bell pepper with the quinoa and black bean mixture, pressing it down gently to fill each pepper evenly.
5. Place the stuffed bell peppers in a baking dish.
6. If desired, sprinkle shredded cheddar cheese over the stuffed peppers for added creaminess and flavor.
7. Bake the stuffed bell peppers in the preheated oven for 25-30 minutes or until the peppers are tender and the cheese is melted and bubbly.
8. Let them cool slightly before serving.

Nutrition (per serving):
- Calories: 350
- Carbohydrates: 40g
- Protein: 15g
- Fat: 15g
- Fiber: 10g

Zucchini Lasagna

- 2 large zucchinis, thinly sliced lengthwise (about 1/4-inch thick)
- 1 pound ground turkey (or beef for a different flavor)
- 2 cups sugar-free tomato sauce
- 1 cup ricotta cheese
- 1 cup shredded mozzarella cheese
- 1/4 cup grated parmesan cheese
- 2 cloves garlic, minced
- 1 tablespoon olive oil
- 1 tablespoon chopped fresh basil
- Salt and pepper to taste

Instructions:

1. Preheat the oven to 375°F (190°C).
2. In a large skillet, heat the olive oil over medium heat. Add the minced garlic and sauté for a minute until fragrant.

3. Add the ground turkey to the skillet until browned and cooked through - season with salt and pepper to taste.

4. Stir in the tomato sauce and chopped basil, and simmer for a few minutes to let the flavors meld.

5. Mix the ricotta cheese and shredded mozzarella cheese in a separate bowl.

6. In a baking dish, layer the zucchini slices to form the lasagna base.

7. Spread a layer of the meat sauce over the zucchini slices.

8. Add a layer of the ricotta and mozzarella cheese mixture to the sauce.

9. Repeat the layers until all the ingredients are used, finishing with a layer of zucchini slices and meat sauce on top.

10. Sprinkle-grated parmesan cheese over the top of the lasagna.

11. Cover the baking dish with foil and bake in the oven for 30 minutes. Remove the foil and

bake for 10-15 minutes until the cheese is melted and bubbly.

12. Let the zucchini lasagna cool slightly before serving.

Nutrition (per serving):

Calories: 400

Carbohydrates: 10g

Protein: 30g

Fat: 25g

Fiber: 3g

Navigating Social Situations and Dining Out on a No-Carb Diet

While following a no-carb diet can bring numerous health benefits, it may also present challenges regarding social gatherings and dining out. This section discusses practical strategies and tips to help you navigate these situations quickly and confidently. From attending parties and family gatherings to dining at restaurants, we'll explore how to stay true to your no-carb lifestyle while enjoying social interactions and delicious meals.

Communicating Your Dietary Preferences

Introduction: Communicating your dietary preferences to friends, family, and hosts is an essential first step in navigating social situations on a no-carb diet. Many people may not be familiar with the concept of a no-carb diet, so explaining your choices in a friendly and informative manner can help set expectations and avoid misunderstandings.

Tips:

- When invited to a social event, consider contacting the host in advance to discuss your dietary restrictions and inquire about the menu. This proactive approach allows the host to accommodate your needs and avoids any last-minute surprises.

- Be polite and grateful for the host's efforts to accommodate your dietary preferences. Expressing gratitude can foster a positive atmosphere and strengthen your relationship with the host.

- Offer to bring a no-carb dish to share with others. This ensures you have a suitable option to enjoy and introduces your friends and family to delicious, no-carb recipes.

Example:

Host: "We would love to have you for dinner this weekend!"

You: "Thank you so much for the kind invitation! I'd love to join you. I wanted to let you know that I'm *currently following a no-carb diet for health reasons. Would it be possible to share the menu in advance so I can plan accordingly? I'm happy to bring a no-carb dish to share with everyone!"*

Navigating Restaurant Menus

Eating out at restaurants can be challenging on a no-carb diet, as many dishes are often rich in carbohydrates. However, you can enjoy a delicious meal that aligns with your dietary goals with a few strategies and modifications.

<u>Tips:</u>

- Study the menu carefully and look for dishes that naturally align with a no-carb lifestyle. Grilled meats, seafood, and salads with protein can be excellent options.
- Don't hesitate to ask questions or request modifications. Most restaurants are accommodating and willing to customize dishes to meet your dietary needs.

- Replace carb-heavy sides, rice or potatoes, with extra vegetables or a salad. Most restaurants are flexible with substitutions.
- Be cautious of hidden carbs in sauces and dressings. Opt for simple oil and vinegar dressings, or ask for sauces on the side to control the portion.

Example:

Waiter: "Are you ready to order?"

You: "Yes, I'd like the grilled chicken breast, but instead of the mashed potatoes, could I have an extra side of steamed vegetables, please? Also, could I have the sauce on the side? I'm following a no-carb diet and want to ensure I stay on track. Thank you!"

Handling Social Pressures

In social settings, you may encounter pressures to indulge in carb-heavy foods or explanations about your dietary choices. Learning how to handle these situations gracefully and confidently will help you stay true to your no-carb lifestyle.

Tips:

- Stay firm but polite when declining carb-laden foods. A simple "No, thank you" or "I'm avoiding carbs for health reasons" is sufficient.
- Focus on the enjoyment of social interactions rather than solely on the food. Engaging in conversations and activities can distract from any potential food-related pressures.
- Remember your motivations for following a no-carb diet and its positive impact on your health. This sense of purpose can bolster your resolve in challenging situations.

Example:

Friend: "Come on, just one slice of cake won't hurt! It's a special occasion."

You: "I appreciate the gesture but am committed to my no-carb diet for health reasons. I'm feeling *great and want to stay on track. Thank you for understanding!"*

Finding No-Carb Options at Social Events

Social events like parties and gatherings often feature carb-heavy finger foods and snacks. However, with some creativity, you can find no-carb options to enjoy without compromising your dietary goals.

Tips:

- Seek protein-based appetizers like deviled eggs, cheese platters, or grilled chicken skewers.
- Load up on low-carb vegetables, such as cucumber slices, bell pepper strips, and cherry tomatoes, while avoiding high-carb dips and sauces.
- If there's a salad bar, create a no-carb salad with leafy greens, protein, nuts, and seeds, using a simple oil and vinegar dressing.
- Focus on the company and conversations rather than constantly grazing on food.

Example:

At a party, you spot a tray of finger foods that all seem carb-heavy. You head to the snack table and choose a few deviled eggs, a small serving of mixed nuts, and fresh vegetable sticks. Throughout the evening, you engage in lively conversations and enjoy the company of friends, not feeling the need to snack constantly.

Conclusion

Embarking on a no-carb journey can be a transformative and empowering experience for your health and well-being. Throughout this guide, we have explored the fundamental principles of a no-carb diet, its benefits, and practical steps to implement this lifestyle successfully. You can tap into many advantages by eliminating or significantly reducing carbohydrates, including better blood sugar control, enhanced weight management, increased energy levels, and improved mental clarity.

Understanding the impact of carbohydrates on your body and learning to distinguish between good and bad carbs is crucial. By prioritizing whole, nutrient-dense foods and avoiding processed and refined carbohydrates, you can ensure your body receives the vital nutrients it needs to thrive. We have delved into the no-carb food list, revealing various delicious and nourishing options to incorporate into your daily meals, from fresh vegetables and healthy fats to protein-rich sources and flavorful herbs and spices.

We discussed the importance of mental and physical preparation to make a smooth transition to a no-carb lifestyle. By setting clear goals, creating a meal plan, and organizing your pantry and kitchen, you set yourself up for success. We have also provided an array of delicious recipes for no-carb breakfasts, lunches, and dinners, proving that you don't have to compromise on taste to eat healthily.

Furthermore, we addressed the benefits and challenges of a no-carb diet and how it can impact your overall health and well-being. By optimizing nutrient intake, stabilizing blood sugar levels, and promoting fat-burning mechanisms, you can experience sustainable and positive changes in your body and mind.

Social situations and dining out can be potential obstacles on a no-carb journey, but we have equipped you with practical strategies to navigate these scenarios easily. From communicating your dietary preferences effectively to finding no-carb options at social events, you can confidently enjoy these experiences while maintaining your commitment to a healthy lifestyle.

In this journey, remember that consistency and self-compassion are essential. It's okay to have occasional deviations if you refocus on your no-carb goals. Embrace the support of friends, family, and online communities that share your dietary choices. Celebrate your progress, big and small, and recognize the positive changes you make for your body and well-being.

As you embark on your no-carb adventure, remember this is a sustainable and fulfilling lifestyle, not a temporary diet. Be patient with yourself and give your body the time it needs to adjust and thrive. Listen to your body's signals and adjust to suit your unique needs.

By incorporating various delicious and nutrient-dense foods, staying mindful of your dietary choices in social situations, and prioritizing your overall well-being, you can embark on a rewarding no-carb journey that brings you closer to your health goals. Remember, a no-carb lifestyle is not about deprivation; it's about nourishing your body with the best possible fuel to lead a vibrant and fulfilling life.

So, embrace the power of no-carb living, and may this journey bring vitality, clarity, and the joy of relishing delicious, wholesome foods. Here's to a healthier, happier you!

Made in the USA
Columbia, SC
01 May 2025

57410577R10043